holy smokes

Inspirational Help for
Kicking the Habit

holy smokes

jean flora glick

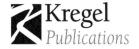
Kregel
Publications

Holy Smokes: Inspirational Help for Kicking the Habit

© 2003 by Jean Flora Glick

Published by Kregel Publications, a division of Kregel, Inc., P.O. Box 2607, Grand Rapids, MI 49501.

Cover design: John M. Lucas

Library of Congress Cataloging-in-Publication Data
Glick, Jean Flora.
Holy smokes: inspirational help for kicking the habit / by Jean Flora Glick.
    p. cm.
Includes bibliographical references.
    1. Tobacco habit—Prevention—Miscellanea. 2. Cigarette habit—Prevention—Miscellanea. 3. Cigarette smokers—Religious life. I. Title.
HV5735.G55   2003
613.85—dc21   2003012162

ISBN 0-8254-2696-0

Printed in the United States of America

03 04 05 06 07 / 5 4 3 2 1

This book is lovingly dedicated
to my husband, John,
to my mother, Pearl Flora Wells,
and to the memory of my dad,
William L. Flora.

Contents

Acknowledgments

I am grateful for the encouragement and support of my prayer partners, Janet Teitsort and Carol Layman. No two friends could be more cherished.

I appreciate the encouragement from my family, Kathy and Mike Hayes; Kim and John Eric Nading; Kerry and Julie Glick; and my beloved grandchildren, Kira Marie and Cameron Glick; Stephanie Glick; Ryan and Robyn Ferguson; Lance and Luke Erb; Aran and Melanie Nading.

I have been blessed to receive insight and illumination from Rev. Sandra Crase, pastor of the Moravian Church on the Morongo Indian Reservation in Banning, California.

I appreciate the prayers of discussion groups in the Evening Women's Bible Study Fellowship class of Columbus, Indiana, and the prayers of Celia Gibson, Teaching Leader.

I am grateful to Florence and Marita Littaurer and the CLASS organization for career coaching seminars and access to publishers.

I am thankful for longtime friends Judy Keene, Veda Eddy, Debbie DeWeese, Shirley Wyant, and Delores Wright who have inspired me in many ways.

A Letter from Jean

Dear Reader,

"My daughter is trying to stop smoking," I told the clerk in the Ark, a local Christian bookstore. "I want an inspirational book that will encourage Kim. What can you suggest?"

The clerk typed in "stop smoking" on her computer. Nothing. She tried several other keywords without success. Finally she said, "I don't find any titles that fit your description."

As I left the store, the clerk called out to me, "If you do find such a book, let me know. I want to buy one for my daughter!"

Having smoked for twenty-four years, my forty-one-year-old daughter Kim has tried repeatedly to overcome her tobacco addiction. Many times I've been her cheerleader as she attempted to quit. In an effort to help her, I've gathered gruesome and tragic stories of deathbed pleas from longtime smokers. I've gathered statistics about the number of people who died annually from lung cancer. Although I shared all these stories and statistics with Kim, she was still hooked.

"Mother, I'm sorry," Kim confided, her face forlorn as a stray kitten. "Those frightful stories about smokers don't do me any good. I know I'm addicted. I know smoking is unhealthy. What I need is something positive to help me through the rough spots."

As I continued to pray about it, I remembered that Kim had always loved letters from me. When she'd lived out of state, I'd written to her daily. I wondered what would happen if I wrote her a daily encouragement letter and included something to make her smile and something tangible as a keepsake.

I decided to give it a try.

Each day, I penned Kim a letter based on Scripture, decorated the stationery and envelope, and tucked in a little reward. Kim began to respond with letters of her own, and over time we compiled the correspondence that became the cornerstone of this book. Our prayer for you as you read is that you too will discover heavenly help to stop smoking.

All my best,
Jean

A Letter from Kim

Dear Reader,

I'm writing this letter at the beginning—before I undertake Mom's program for quitting cigarettes.

I am forty-one years old, and I've smoked for twenty-four years. I'm married and have an eighteen-year-old daughter, Stephanie. I'm an artist, having completed three years of art school, although I supplement our family income by cleaning houses. And I'm addicted to smoking—a statement that's hard to admit but true. For the past four years, I've tried periodically and unsuccessfully to quit. The longest I've been without a cigarette, until now, has been two weeks.

Becoming a nicotine addict was not something I wanted for myself—it just happened, puff by puff. When I was young, Dad smoked, and I was always afraid he would die and leave me. So, in fourth grade, I started a letter-writing campaign to get Dad to quit. His smoking didn't seem to bother my older sister, Kathy, or my younger brother, Kerry. But for me the campaign became an obsession, my mission.

I hid letters under Dad's pillow, left notes in his pickup truck, even tucked messages in his newspaper. I drew pictures, wrote speeches. For four years, no results! Then, much to my surprise, when I was in seventh grade, my father quit smoking cold turkey. Without telling us. When I noticed he didn't have a cigarette dangling out of his mouth, I was so proud of him!

The summer before my senior year of high school, I was a rebellious teenager. I didn't like my father much then. He made rules I had to follow! One way I could hurt him was to smoke. So I did. Once I was hooked, I became ashamed of my nicotine addiction. I don't allow photos or videos of me smoking, and I never smoke in front of Mom or Dad.

This time, however, my approach to quitting is different. Mom has promised to write me a daily letter of encouragement. I'm praying, really praying. And I'm taking a step of faith. As the Reverend Charles Stanley wrote in *The Wonderful Spirit-Filled Life*, "Faith is the Holy Spirit's signal to go into action." I'm taking that first step, but I'm very afraid of failing again. . . .

Giving it my best,
Kim

1

The Battle Is the Lord's

Dear Kim,

You can be encouraged by David, the shepherd boy who stood strong as he faced nine-foot-tall Goliath. This giant warrior wore 125 pounds of armor and carried a massive spear—its iron point alone weighed 15 pounds. With no armor, five smooth stones, and faith in God, David defied Goliath, saying, "All those gathered here will know that it is not by sword or spear that the LORD saves; for the battle is the LORD's, and he will give all of you into our hands" (1 Sam. 17:47).

"Do not be afraid or discouraged because of this vast army. For the battle is not yours, but God's" (2 Chron. 20:15).

Like David, you have a choice. You can give in to Goliath or turn the battle over to the Lord. You'll make the right choice, I know. I'm cheering for you, Kim. The score's going to be Kim: 1; Goliath: 0. You're the winner! Pray a prayer of surrender to God and start by kneeling when you pray.

Love,
Mom

Hey Mom,

Yes, it's God's battle not mine! I know that the Lord who delivered me from depression a few years ago is the same Lord who will deliver me from my smoking addiction.

I'm weak and cannot fight the battle without Him.

I must confess that I woke up and smoked a cigarette without

even remembering that this was *the day I was going to quit!* I was
so discouraged. . . . That is how ingrained the smoking habit is
in me!

Well great, I've blown it already, I thought. I wanted to start
with a clean slate, not with a cigarette. When I've tried to quit
other times, I've tried hypnotism, reducing the number of cigarettes I smoke each day, quitting cold turkey, and wearing a
nicotine patch. But I've never tried to lean on the Holy Spirit
for this. And I never thought of letting the Lord fight my battle.

I decided I'd put on a nicotine patch and started praying on
my knees as you suggested: "Please change me, Lord, to who
You want me to be. I know our relationship is harmed, and
You can't use me now. Forgive me, Father, for I have damaged
Your creation, my body, by exposing it to twenty-four years of
smoking. Have mercy on me, Lord Jesus, and deliver me from
this smoking addiction. Change me. Mold me. Use me. In Jesus'
name, Amen."

Love you,
Kim

Smile Break

When you get to your wit's end, you'll find God lives
there.

—Elizabeth Yates

My Journal Page

Prayer

Lord, I surrender my addiction to You. I am helpless, but Holy Spirit, You are the Helper. Keep me strong this day; help me to remain firm and steadfast. Let me rest in You, Lord, knowing the battle is Yours and victory is mine. In Jesus' name, Amen.

Action

Kneel as you pray.

2

Scripture in My Pocket

Dear Kim,

Memorizing Bible verses started for me with a little card calendar that our church gave me at the first of the year. I placed the card on the car dash and noticed it every time I drove. It advised, "Cast all your anxiety on him because he cares for you" (1 Peter 5:7).

That was helpful. It made me hungry for more daily Scripture. So I started writing verses on index cards and carrying them in my purse.

I remember the day I lost my job at the museum. My supervisor called me to her office one Thursday and said, "Jean, we're making your job part time with no insurance benefits. You think about it and give me an answer on Monday."

I knew I wasn't going to commute an hour one way for a part-time job with no insurance. On Friday, my supervisor was out of the office. I wanted to say good-bye to the museum volunteers and my coworkers without their knowing it was my last day. In my skirt pocket I carried a card with 2 Timothy 1:7: "For God did not give us a spirit of timidity [fear], but a spirit of power, of love and of self-discipline." All that day I told each person in a roundabout way how I'd enjoyed working with her or him and gave each one a hug. I knew I'd probably never see them again. They suspected nothing. After work I was the last to leave. I cleaned out my desk and office of personal belongings. Having that Scripture in my pocket got me through the day.

Love and hugs,
Mom

Hi Mom,

I got up and had no coffee! I said to Stephanie, "How can I give up two things at once?"

No coffee, no smoking—it's too much.

So off I whizzed to the convenience store for a French vanilla cappuccino to go. Outside the store, I spotted an ashtray—a powerful urge to scavenge a cigarette butt gripped me . . . but I resisted.

When I read your letter about your last day working at the museum and carrying the Scripture in your pocket, the thought of your saying a secret good-bye brought a lump to my throat. It was a sad ending to your job, yet there was a victory there, too.

Today I chose to memorize the Scripture verse that's written on the cover of my journal, "The LORD is faithful to all His promises and loving toward all he has made" (Ps. 145:13).

This morning, which began with little promise, turned into a better-than-okay day. I felt spiritually high. I felt prayers surrounding me, and it was amazingly easy not to smoke. This is not the norm, I know. Although the full-strength nicotine patch made a welt on my arm, I'm going to get past that. Over and over this thought popped in my mind, "Remember the blessings, Kim. Remember the blessings."

At peace,
Your daughter

Smile Break

The Bible that is falling apart usually belongs to someone who isn't.

—Source Unknown

My Journal Page

Prayer

Heavenly Father, help me to memorize Your words so I can carry them with me. Help me to cast all my anxiety upon You. In Your Son's name, Amen.

Action

Memorize a Scripture that will help you.

_____
_____
_____
_____
_____
_____
_____
_____
_____
_____
_____
_____
_____
_____
_____

3

You Are Special

Dearest Kim,

You need to remember every day, in every way, how very important you are to God and to me. Whether you smoke or not, we love you. But remember how proud of yourself you'll be when you beat this addiction. Your spirit-lifter for today is this poem by Marcia Krugh Leaser that I found in a magazine.

Self-Worth

The only eyes you need to use
    When looking at yourself
Are eyes full of forgiveness—
    Putting guilt upon a shelf.

God did not die for only those
    Who live life perfectly.
He gave His life for everyone
    Namely . . . you and me.

You may not feel you're worthy
    Of God's death upon a cross—
You've sinned too much for His dear blood
    To pay that high a cost.

But Jesus came for you, my friend.
    You are worth the pain He knew.

He would have come, suffered and died
If the world contained . . . just you.

*You're special, so do something special for yourself today.
Mom*

Hello Mama Dear,

You say I am special to you and God, but I feel like a worm. It has been a terrible day. I took off my 21 mg patch to shower, put on another patch, and I must have double dosed on nicotine. I felt sick, so I tore off the patch and decided I'd go cold turkey. No patch. No cigarettes.

When I went to the grocery, I began to cry—without warning. It was embarrassing! There I was shopping for milk and eggs, and I lost it. I started bawling and could not stop. Other shoppers must have thought, *Who died?* The guy behind the meat counter, Bobby Garrison, quit the habit and has been smoke free for a year. I asked him what to do, and he replied, "Don't give up. You can beat this."

Back home, I was a witch. I said to Stephanie, "Look close! This is what the nicotine monster looks like. It's panic time—put me in a padded cell."

John tiptoed around trying to stay out of my way. Finally, he mumbled, "I'm going outside to do some yard work." As he left, he said, "Help us out. Give us a break. Smoke a cigarette!"

Mom, you suggested I do something special for myself. What I decided to do was take a relaxing bubble bath with candles lit. Then I looked in the tub; it was as grungy as the dungeon where the Count of Monte Cristo was imprisoned. So, on my hands and knees, I angrily scrubbed the tub—ready to explode like a firecracker.

At 11:30 P.M., I scuttled to the basement for a smoke. I felt like Pigpen in a Charlie Brown cartoon—engulfed in a nasty cloud of odor. When I walked upstairs, Stephanie caught me and from her look I knew she knew. "Yes," I told her, "I smoked a cigarette, and it tasted good!"

I'm wondering why God is torturing me when I've prayed and taken the initiative to quit this awful habit.

Trapped in ugly thoughts,
Kim

Smile Break

I was pure as the driven snow but I drifted.

—Mae West

My Journal Page

Prayer

Lamb of God, thank You for suffering and dying on the cross for me. Thank You for eternal life. Your sacrifice makes me feel loved and so special.

Action

Do something special for yourself today.

4

Lead Me Not into Temptation

My darling daughter,

You're angry because you think God has tempted you. Wrong thinking! According to James 1:13–14, "When tempted, no one should say, 'God is tempting me.' For God cannot be tempted by evil, nor does he tempt anyone; but each one is tempted when, by his own evil desire, he is dragged away and enticed."

Instead of blaming God, you need to take responsibility for your choice to begin smoking years ago. Then realize that God created you and He loves you. Consider the homeless kitten that appeared at your door recently. Hearing that pitiful cry, you opened the door to your heart. You lavished love on that kitty even though it had fleas, runny eyes, and ear mites.

Remember, God loves you as you are. Read 1 John 4:16: "And so we know and rely on the love God has for us. God is love. Whoever lives in love lives in God, and God in him."

Throughout the day today, picture yourself snuggled in God's embrace, loved like an abandoned kitten. Remind yourself of three ways you know God loves you.

As ever,
Mom

Dear Mama,

Comparing my love for the homeless kitty with God's love for me—I like that! I know God loves me because . . .

1. He sent His son Jesus to die for my sins—my willful sins—so I could be saved.
2. I can feel His love through the Holy Spirit in me.
3. He has blessed me by protecting me many times over the past years.

I've discovered that the 21 mg nicotine patch is too strong for me. . . . I've switched to 14 mg patches. Also, I allow myself five bad moments a day. That is, when the urge for a cigarette becomes fierce I say, "Kim, hold on . . . wait a little longer. . . . You can be strong a few more minutes." This mental chitchat helps. I've noticed that struggling with this habit is a mental as well as a physical game.

I'll add a fourth way I know God loves me: As I worked in the yard, a kitten hopped under our hedge and was by my side all day. This evening, my neighbor begged me to adopt the kitten. I hesitated, because I already have Puff, Teesha, and Tigger. But I couldn't resist—I didn't want this kitten taken to the Humane Society. It's funny—God always seems to send me a kitty to help me through my toughest times. I've named my new friend who now lives with us Farley. This precious, adorable, huggable fluff ball has to be God's love gift to me. I wanted to celebrate Farley's arrival with a cigarette, but I resisted.

Meow, meow,
Kim

Smile Break

Cats are smarter than dogs. You can't get eight cats to pull a sled through snow.

—Jeff Valdez

My Journal Page

Prayer

Heavenly Father, hold me close today, keeping me in Your care. I know this for sure: I am loved, I am loved, I am loved.

Action

Recall three ways you know God loves you.

_____

_____

_____

_____

_____

_____

_____

_____

_____

_____

_____

_____

_____

_____

_____

_____

_____

5

Your Wake-up Call

Dear Kim,

What are your first words as you wake up each morning? Are they "Good Lord, it's morning!" Or do you say, "Good morning, Lord!"

As my eyes pop open, I like to greet the morning by thinking, *"This is the day the Lord has made; let us rejoice and be glad in it"* (Ps. 118:24).

I've been told that Reverend Ray Stedman, the late pastor of Peninsula Bible Church in Palo Alto, California, used to start each morning with this wake-up routine. He reminded himself:

1. I'm made in the image of God, with an ability to relate and respond to God.
2. I'm filled with the Spirit of God, who is at work in me through the problems and pressures I have each day.
3. I'm part of the plan of God. God is working out all things to a great and final purpose on earth. Therefore, what I do today has significance and meaning.

He said that thinking of ourselves in this way gives us "confidence without conceit."

So greet each new day in confidence, knowing you're made in the image of God, you're filled with the Holy Spirit, and your day has meaning and purpose.

Remain in His care,
Mom

Mother Dear,

I like Reverend Stedman's wake up routine. I'm definitely not a morning person. It's important for me to put on the patch first thing—even before my cup of coffee—or I'll smoke. In the morning, since the patch has been off all night, my nicotine level is low; I'm almost in a panic.

What has helped me immensely is a decision made a year ago—when I tried to stop smoking and failed. I made myself *not* smoke in the house; my smoking area became our basement. Now the house is smoke free for Stephanie. Plus, it's not very pleasurable puffing away in a dank, mildewed basement.

I'm struggling with the 14 mg patch. It doesn't fully stop my craving for a cigarette. Smoking is like having a concrete block hanging around my neck.

When I worked in retail, I could tell every smoker who came in my department. Each one reeked of smoke, looked older than her age, and I realized, "Holy smokes, that's how I look and smell to others."

When I started smoking at seventeen, I never thought that time would fast forward to forty-one. I never thought I'd have to suffer the consequences of twenty-four years of addiction. I remember the first cigarette I smoked. It was nasty. But soon I was hooked. Part of it was peer pressure, and a huge part of it was rebellion.

When I was younger, I tried quitting cold turkey. That lasted a few days until I became such a monster I couldn't recognize myself. Oh, I long for the day when I'm smoke free.

Hanging by a thread,
Kim

Smile Break

A cigarette company is coming out with a mint that has as much nicotine as a cigarette. Great. Now we can die from secondhand breath as well. The mints are called Life Takers.

—Jay Leno

My Journal Page

Prayer

Holy Spirit, I pray Psalm 5:3, "In the morning, O LORD, you hear my voice; in the morning I lay my requests before you and wait in expectation."

Action

Take a walk when you're tempted to smoke; jot down your thoughts.

6

Straight Arrow or Zigzag?

Dear Kim,

You're wavering, and I sympathize with your frustration. I recall a time when my intentions were good, but they went awry. I wanted to send my friend Janet a get-well card. Grabbing the card from the kitchen table, I noticed a stain on the tablecloth. *Better put that in the washer,* I thought.

When I tossed the tablecloth in the washer, I saw I had only a half load. *Better retrieve more dirty laundry from the bedroom clothes hamper.* In the bedroom, I noticed our unmade bed. *Okay, I'd better make the bed before I forget.* As I was straightening the sheets and pulling up the blanket, I heard the water running in the washer. *Oh my, I'd better get the rest of that dirty laundry.* Gathering the dirty clothes from the hamper, I zipped to the washer. *Yikes!*—there sat my tennis shoes without shoestrings. *Oh yes, those new shoelaces are in my purse, which I left in the car in the garage.*

As I rummaged in the car, the phone rang. Hurrying to the kitchen with my purse, I answered the phone. It was a friend who wanted an e-mail address—which was in my office . . . upstairs. I transferred over to my office phone. While I was looking up the e-mail address, *Gee–I see my wastebasket overflows.* Hurrying downstairs with the trash, I heard the UPS man tap at the front door. When I opened the door, he gave me an odd look. *Hasn't he ever seen a woman with tennis shoes in her right hand, a trash bag in her left hand, and a purse handle clenched in her teeth?*

"I'm sending a card to Janet," I mumbled. He rolled his eyes and gently closed the door.

Kim, I've discovered that some people are straight arrows,

whereas others zigzag, losing sight of their target. It's the same spiritually. Some go straight to their daily devotions and prayer with God. Others get sidetracked. Proverbs 4:25, 27 says, "Let your eyes look straight ahead, fix your gaze directly before you. . . . Do not swerve to the right or the left; keep your foot from evil." Are you a straight-arrow believer—or a zigzagger who leaves the bed half made, your sneakers without laces, and the downstairs phone off the hook?

Do a load of laundry. Send a card to a friend.

Holy Smokes! Stay focused on Jesus,
Mom

Hi Mom,

Gee whiz—do a load of laundry? No way! I already do laundry every day, sometimes five loads. That's what led me to smoking! Seriously, though, I did write a note to April. I am so much like you, Mom. I'm a zigzag person who gets sidetracked, and I don't think it's something I can change. (Some things are meant to be.)

Still, I felt as low as a junkyard dog today. And just as mean . . . grrrr!

This afternoon, I craved a cigarette so fiercely I wanted to bristle and growl and grovel!

Throughout the day, I sent "arrow prayers" to God to stay sane. This restrained me from barking! Around five o'clock, I ripped off my patch and smoked two cigarettes.

I almost bit John's ears when he got home from work and innocently asked, "How's it going today?"

Tonight I may even howl at the moon!

Love ya,
Kim

Smile Break

Tobacco companies will stop at nothing to win the tobacco wars. Now their scientists are saying some of the smoking research data is no longer valid because the rats have to step outside their mazes to smoke.

—Dennis Miller

My Journal Page

Prayer

Holy God, help me be a straight arrow, focusing on You.

Action

Do a load of laundry (at your discretion). Send a card to a friend. Don't get sidetracked.

_____

_____

_____

_____

_____

_____

_____

_____

_____

_____

_____

_____

_____

_____

_____

_____

_____

7

Begin Again

Dearest Kim,

Our God is a God of second chances. A God of third chances. A God of forgiveness.

You are no doubt discouraged that you've relapsed, and now you'll need to put on your patches and begin again. This poem by Louise Fletcher Tarkington tugged at my heart:

> I wish there were
> Some wonderful place
> Called the Land of Beginning Again,
> Where all our mistakes
> And all our heartaches
> And all our poor selfish grief
> Could be dropped like
> A shabby old coat at the door
> And never put on again.

So, Kim dear, shed your shabby coat and begin again. Consider King David and what he learned. Although it was the desire of David's heart to build a magnificent house for God, he realized that God's plan was for Solomon, David's son, to build the temple in Jerusalem. King David ordered all the leaders of Israel to help Solomon. In 1 Chronicles 22:16, David says to Solomon, "Now begin the work, and the LORD be with you."

I encourage you to start over and rebuild your "holy temple"— your body. And may the Lord be with you.

Love,
Mom

Dear Mom,

I can't do it. I can't begin again. When I stop smoking, it is a full-time endeavor to concentrate on not smoking. It's too hard.

This will shock you—and I'm sorry—but I don't care if I do get cancer. Then my struggle on earth will be over and I can rest in paradise. I suppose if I did learn tomorrow I had cancer, I would then want desperately to live.

I smoke because:

1. My life is boring. Cleaning houses is mindless, routine work. I smoke to reward myself.
2. There is no support for me—my husband and friends smoke and no one (except you) believes I can quit.
3. Some people are joyful and self-confident. I feel worthless and guilty—smoking eases the pain.
4. People pity me and my bad habit. My cigarettes comfort me.

Just write me off as a lost cause, Mom. I'm a loser.

Sadly,
Kim

Smile Break

Loser: an innocent bystander who gets killed after a battle by an unexploded shell and then has his name spelled wrong in the newspapers.

—Colin Bowles,
The Wit's Dictionary

My Journal Page

Prayer

Holy Spirit, enable and empower me to begin again. I thank
You for another chance to rebuild my holy temple, keeping
it clean and pure as my act of worship. Amen.

Action

Write down your two greatest concerns as you begin again
and what will be your two greatest rewards as you start over.

_____

_____

_____

_____

_____

_____

_____

_____

_____

_____

_____

_____

_____

_____

_____

_____

_____

8

You're Not a Loser

Hello dear Kim,

You may think you're a loser—I don't. In Matthew 17, the disciples tried to heal a boy possessed by a demon. They failed. When the boy was brought to Jesus, He rebuked the demon and the boy was healed instantly. Later, the disciples came to Jesus in private and asked, "Why couldn't we drive it out?"

Jesus replied, "Because you have so little faith. I tell you the truth, if you have faith as small as a mustard seed, you can say to this mountain, 'Move from here to there' and it will move. Nothing will be impossible for you" (Matt. 17:19–20).

You lack faith. I know a Kim who believed so much in God's power that your unswerving faith moved a mountain. Two years ago, you hosted that exchange student from Ecuador. Despite her radiant smile, which was warm enough to melt an icicle, Adriana Serrano hid a sorrow that she eventually confided to you: "My sister, Tania, is in very bad health."

Tania was dying of kidney failure brought on by lupus complications. She spent six hours daily giving herself kidney dialysis. Adriana's family had sold their car and furniture for medicine for Tania; a kidney transplant was beyond their resources. As Adriana's host mother, you prayed, "Lord, help me to help Tania."

You organized a teen dance as a fund-raiser; you appealed to local churches. You prayed; you left the rest to God. Two months later, a miraculous $10,000 had been raised and wired to Ecuador. Tania's brother had a 75 percent compatible kidney that he offered. Surgery was performed, and six weeks later Tania was home from the hospital with a new kidney.

A dying young woman in Ecuador now plays volleyball and

attends college—her life restored by your firm faith that the impossible was possible. Believe, Kim. Only believe.

Mom

Dear Mother,

Thank you for believing in me when I can't even believe in myself. Today I learned a shocking fact: After one hundred thousand cigarettes, a smoker plays Russian roulette. At any time, lung cancer can manifest itself.

As a smoker for twenty-four years, I've reached that quota. Now, as I place a cigarette in my mouth, the thought whaps me, "Is this the *one* that will trigger lung cancer?"

How did this awful habit begin? When I was fourteen, I remember my friend Lisa's mom smoked. When I was at Lisa's house, we filched cigarettes from her mom's stash. The first cigarette made me sick and dizzy. It was like licking a dog food dish. Nasty!

Then, the summer before my senior year in high school, I started smoking one or two cigarettes each weekend. At parties, I smoked one or two here and there. Soon those cigarettes didn't taste foul. It got me! I was addicted.

Now a gremlin with claws has me in its clutches. I want control over this addiction, but I don't have it.

Holding a smoking gun,
Kim

Smile Break

What are cigarettes?
Answer: Killers who travel in packs.

—Mary Ott

My Journal Page

Prayer

Lord Jesus, increase my faith so I can move this impossible mountain of addiction and stop smoking.

Action

Reflect on your faith and believe.

9

Daughter of the King

Dear Kim,

You have me puzzled. Why do you have such low self-esteem? God has given you a tremendous talent—you are an artist. I still puff up with pride remembering your one-woman art show at the Southern Indiana Center for the Arts. Your paintings, wood carvings, and metal sculptures filled two rooms! You painted the background for your church's Tour of Bethlehem; you've created dazzling after-prom decorations; you've thrilled Rhonda by painting a forty-foot-long by twelve-foot-high mural on her outside retaining wall.

You're a compassionate person, the hero of many stray and abandoned kittens and other assorted animals and birds. You can organize clutter like nobody's business; four of your former bosses have applauded your ability to organize massive amounts of paper clutter.

Most importantly, you are royalty. That's right, you are the daughter of the King! When you gave your heart to Jesus as a fourteen-year-old, you came into your inheritance. Romans 8:16–17 says, "The Spirit himself testifies with our spirit that we are God's children. Now if we are children, then we are heirs—heirs of God and co-heirs with Christ."

John 1:12 further assures us, "Yet to all who received him, to those who believed in his name, he gave the right to become children of God." According to Ephesians 5:8–10, "For you were once darkness, but now you are light in the Lord. Live as children of light (for the fruit of the light consists in all goodness, righteousness and truth) and find out what pleases the Lord." It would please our Sovereign Lord, I believe, if you would claim your inheritance and live like the true daughter of the King that you are.

Love you much,
Mom

Dear Mom,

You're right. . . . I am living like a chimney sweep instead of claiming my royalty as a daughter of the King. You ask why I place such a low value on myself. . . .

I've believed the negative messages that have played and replayed in my mind. Messages such as, "Art is play—not something for grown-ups, not something you can have as a career." Where did such a thought come from? I don't know—maybe an art teacher, maybe a friend. Wherever it originated, I grabbed it and branded it in my brain.

A second negative tape repeats: "You're weak; you've tried to quit smoking before. You never follow through. You'll fail."

Another negative voice claims, "You can't quit smoking, because your husband and your closest friends smoke." Well, when I shine a spotlight on that lie, I see that it's an excuse.

In my devotions, I discovered a few verses that made me chuckle, because once again God had a PS to add to your letter. It's Philippians 2:14–16, "Do everything without complaining or arguing, so that you may become blameless and pure, children of God without fault in a crooked and depraved generation, in which you shine like stars in the universe as you hold out the word of life."

Now excuse me as I visualize myself shining like a star (smoke free).

I'll be a sunbeam for Jesus,
Kim

Smile Break

In the Bible, the words "Fear not" can be found 365 times; once for every day of the year.

—Catherine Hall, *More Holy Humor*

My Journal Page

Prayer

King of kings, help me to live as Your child of light today.

Action

Visualize yourself as a nonsmoker, instead of a smoker who is quitting.

_____
_____
_____
_____
_____
_____
_____
_____
_____
_____
_____
_____
_____
_____
_____
_____

10

Winning the Race

My dear Kim,

You are running a race of perseverance. Each day you are closer to your goal. This reminds me of when I was fourteen and wanted to enter the Hope Heritage Day's bike race. However, several of my friends who had their driver's permit hooted, "Being on a bike is baby stuff. Why don't you just hop on your bike and lead the parade? Now that would be cool!" So I wrestled with the choice: be accepted by my peers or be ridiculed.

I entered the race and told no one. However, my friend Georgia got suspicious. When she learned what I was doing, she said, "If you're silly enough to do it, I will too." Then Wilma thought she might as well race also. Great! With their competition, I might not win!

As determined as if I were training for the Olympics, I practiced every day. Because the route was along Jackson Street, it would be a cinch—two blocks and all downhill! Still, I left nothing to chance. I trained with a vengeance.

Race day came. The starter whistle blew. I tore off like a tornado, pumping and pedaling, never coasting for a second. At the finish line, I didn't brake. Onlookers were amazed as I whizzed by at warp speed. Actually, a straw-bale barricade a block past the finish line stopped my momentum. "You blew us away," Georgia and Wilma wailed. "You rode like you were strapped to a rocket."

Red-faced and breathless, I accepted my prize. A crisp five-dollar bill. Even today when I'm discouraged, wearied, or tempted to quit, I remember how perseverance won a bike race. And victory was sweet! Hebrews 12:1 tells us, "Let us throw off everything that hinders and the sin that so easily entangles, and let us run with perseverance the race marked out for us."

Be encouraged to keep going, Kim. Ah-h-h-h, victory will be sweet.

You can win this race,
Mom

Dearest Mom,

Makes me laugh to think of you racing like a rocket to win that race and capture five dollars. What I'm learning is that my race to quit smoking is not all downhill! This race is definitely hilly—lots of ups and downs.

One thing that hinders me is not knowing someone else who is going through the same battle as I am—someone who wants to quit smoking too. Secondly, I need someone (besides you) who can hold me accountable. That's why I'm joining Freedom From Smoking, a wellness program offered at the local hospital and sponsored by the American Lung Association.

I've enrolled in the program; it's a seven-session class.

Moving on,
Kim

Smile Break

Life is like a ten-speed bicycle. Most of us have gears we never use.

—Charles M. Schulz

My Journal Page

Prayer

Wonderful Counselor, help me throw off all that hinders me today. Let me not give in to temptation.

Action

Name two things that hinder you and what you can do to overcome them.

_____

_____

_____

_____

_____

_____

_____

_____

_____

_____

_____

_____

_____

_____

_____

_____

_____

_____

11

Benefits of Not Smoking

Dearest Kim,

As soon as you quit smoking, you will receive benefits. According to the American Lung Association, as soon as you snuff out that last cigarette, your body will begin a series of physiological changes. Here's the timeline:

- Within eight hours: "Smoker's breath" disappears. Carbon monoxide level in your blood drops, and oxygen level rises to normal.
- Within twenty-four hours: Chance of heart attack decreases.
- Within forty-eight hours: Nerve endings start to regroup. Ability to taste and smell improves.
- Within three days: Breathing is easier.
- Within two to three months: Circulation improves. Walking becomes easier. Lung capacity increases up to 30 percent.
- Within one to nine months: Sinus congestion and shortness of breath decrease. Cilia that sweep debris from your lungs grow back. Energy increases.
- Within one year: Excess risk of coronary heart disease is half that of a person who still smokes.
- Within two years: Heart attack risk drops to near normal.
- Within five years: Lung cancer death rate for an average former pack-a-day smoker decreases by almost half. Stroke risk is reduced. Risk of mouth, throat, and esophageal cancer is half that of a smoker.
- Within ten years: Lung cancer death rate is similar to

that of a person who does not smoke. The precancerous cells are replaced.

- Within fifteen years: Risk of coronary heart disease is the same as a person who has never smoked.[1]

Write down three benefits of your own that you'll have when you quit smoking.

Lovingly,
Mom

Dear Mother,
These are the benefits (I can do better than name three) I can visualize from not smoking:

1. I will breathe better.
2. I'll have renewed energy—from more oxygen.
3. I will be able to go all day without needing a nap.
4. A clear cough—not a phlegmy cough.
5. No worry over having bad breath.
6. Stamina like nonsmoking people have.
7. Absence of chest pains.
8. Fewer jaw pains from TMJ, aggravated by smoking.
9. Food will taste better.
10. Can get my teeth bleached (they're amazingly yellow).

With benefits like these, I wonder: *Why am I smoking?*

Puzzled,
Kim

Smile Break

Chain smokers get rusty lungs.

—Anne Olivier

My Journal Page

Prayer

Help me, heavenly Healer, to envision how healthy my body, mind, and soul will be when You help me overcome this addiction.

Action

Write down three benefits you'll have when you quit smoking.

_____

_____

_____

_____

_____

_____

_____

_____

_____

_____

_____

_____

_____

_____

_____

_____

_____

_____

12

My Spiritual Blessings

Dear Kim,

You've learned about the health benefits of not smoking. Now Psalm 103:2–5 summarizes the spiritual blessings that God gives you:

> Praise the LORD, O my soul,
> and forget not all his benefits—
> who forgives all your sins
> and heals all your diseases,
> who redeems your life from the pit
> and crowns you with love and compassion,
> who satisfies your desires with good things
> so that your youth is renewed like the eagle's.

You can rejoice, knowing that these benefits are yours because God says so. Imagine seeing your strength renewed until you can soar like an eagle.

Start a gratitude journal. Each day number your blessings; see how quickly you get to one hundred.

Fly high,
Mom

Dear Mama,

Thank you for reminding me of these holy benefits that accompany the health benefits.

Page one of my gratitude journal would include these blessings:

First, God's grace—He loves even a sinner like me. This gives me assurance and confidence. Second, my belief in Jesus Christ means eternal life. Third, the Holy Spirit abides in me and guides me. Fourth, Jesus is my Intercessor in heaven; Jesus prays for me. A fifth blessing is that I have no fear of death—I know my next home will be a heavenly one. Knowing this, I have the sixth blessing—peace about eternity with my Lord.

Sometimes I think it would be much easier to fly away to heaven and leave this old world of struggles and stress. In heaven, my spiritual body would be free of smoking.

Enjoying this thought,
Kim

Smile Break

There is nothing more miserable in the world than to arrive in Paradise and look like your passport photo.

—Erma Bombeck,
More Holy Hilarity

My Journal Page

Prayer

Sovereign Lord, thank You for satisfying my desires with good things.

Action

Start a gratitude journal. Number your blessings; see how quickly you get to one hundred.

_____

_____

_____

_____

_____

_____

_____

_____

_____

_____

_____

_____

_____

_____

_____

_____

13

Gardening with God

Dearest Daughter,

Francis Bacon said, "God Almighty first planted a garden. And, indeed it is the purest of human pleasures."

You once told me early one spring, "Mom, I've already bought seeds for my garden. There's something about working in the sunshine and feeling the soil in my hands that is healing, that makes me feel whole."

Yes, in our garden of life, our words and actions broadcast a message. Every day, I sow seeds. Sometimes they are seeds of anger, envy, resentment, pride, selfishness, rebellion.

Other times I sow patience, kindness, love, and faith in my Lord. As I study the Bible, I become more deeply rooted in His Word. Prayer provides the nutrients for my growth; yet the Gardener of our souls is ultimately responsible. As 1 Corinthians 3:7–9 says, "So neither he who plants nor he who waters is anything, but only God, who makes things grow. The man who plants and the man who waters have one purpose, and each will be rewarded according to his own labor. For we are God's fellow workers; you are God's field, God's building."

What are you growing in your garden today? How can you garden with God?

Love,
Mom

Mother Dear,

Today, I wanted to vent every emotion. I knew I was grouchy and not fit to be around another human. I went to Wheatfields, a natural arts learning center, where I was supposed to clean the farmhouse. My friend Pam said, "Kim, we need work done in the garden more than we need the place cleaned."

Working outdoors was a relief. I took my aggravation out on the weeds. No one was there but me and the dirt. Great! I got on my hands and knees. I yanked and pulled and uprooted. In my torment, I thought of how Jesus must have felt when he was tempted in the desert—His pain. Except He was innocent; I'm suffering the consequences from sinful choices.

I got so involved in weeding that I never even wanted a cigarette all afternoon.

Pleased,
Kim

PS I also got so involved that I didn't put on sunscreen and sunburned my shoulders. For one day I charred my back instead of my lungs!

Smile Break

A garden is a thing of beauty and a job forever.
—Anonymous

My Journal Page

Prayer

Master Gardener, let love, patience, kindness, and faith grow in me.

Action

Garden with God today.

14

Kissable Lips

Dear Kim,

A few more reasons to quit smoking: fewer wrinkles, brighter skin, nicer nails, and kissable lips. Dr. Kathy Fields, a dermatologist at the University of California in San Francisco, reports that quitting smoking can take years off your appearance.

Dr. Fields says the research shows that people who smoke more than fifty packs per year are 4.7 times more likely to be wrinkled than nonsmokers. Of course, quitting smoking won't make old wrinkles disappear, but it will help prevent many new wrinkles from forming. Because smoking gives skin a yellowish appearance, shortly after you quit your skin will begin to become rosier.

What about your fingernails? Because smoking decreases blood flow by 30 percent or more, smokers' nails don't grow as fast or as strong as those of nonsmokers. When a person stops smoking, circulation increases. This results in healthier, more beautiful nails.

Now, those lips! Smoking can dry out your lips as much as bad winter weather can. Give up cigarettes and your lips will be more moist—perfect for smooching. As Dr. Fields points out, when it comes to your health, "Kissing is so much better than smoking."[1]

Psalm 63:3–4 suggests how you can use your kissable lips: "Because your love is better than life, my lips will glorify you. I will praise you as long as I live, and in your name I will lift up my hands."

May you grow to be as beautiful as God intended you to be when He first thought of you!

Why not treat yourself to a facial or a manicure?

Mom

Dear Mom,

John would no doubt appreciate my having more kissable lips!

In addition to luscious lips, I've been thinking of important reasons why I want to stop smoking (from my Freedom from Smoking class):

1. I want to stop smoking because it creates barriers in my relationship with the Lord and my family.
2. I want to stop smoking because I feel ashamed, and smoking robs me of my self-esteem and self-confidence.
3. I want to stop smoking because smoking controls all aspects of my life. I want to be free of the chains of addiction.
4. I want to stop smoking because I am tired of being tired and not having enough energy.
5. I want to stop smoking because I do not want to suffer an agonizing death from lung cancer.
6. I want to stop smoking because it will kill me. I won't be one of the lucky ones who can smoke until they are eighty or ninety.
7. I want to stop smoking so I'll live long for my daughter's sake.

What I like about this wellness program is that it's an additional encouragement that helps me believe I *really* can quit. It's highly recommended that we reward ourselves when we do have a smoke-free day. I think a facial or manicure definitely fits the "reward" category.

Hugs,
Kim

Smile Break

I kissed my first woman and smoked my first cigarette on the same day; I have never had time for tobacco since.

—Arturo Toscanini

My Journal Page

Prayer

Gracious God, my lips praise You for Your mercy and abiding love.

Action

Treat yourself to a facial or a manicure.

_____

_____

_____

_____

_____

_____

_____

_____

_____

_____

_____

_____

_____

_____

_____

_____

_____

_____

_____

15

Armed for Battle

Dear Kim,

I picture you dressed for the day wearing your cat T-shirt
and jeans (although, for the war against addiction that you're
fighting, you need tougher armor).

As I pray for you today, I'll envision you clad in your battle
fatigues. Ephesians 6:10 says, "Be strong in the Lord and in his
mighty power."

Ephesians 6:11–18 explains how you can put on the full armor of God and stand firm. Remember that salvation is your
helmet; your breastplate is righteousness. Buckle on the belt of
truth. Your weapon is what the Spirit gives you—that is, words
that come from God.

Let the sandals on your feet be the gospel of peace so you
will have firm footing. Finally, lift up the great shield of faith
that enables you to quench the flaming arrows of the Evil One.

Draw me a sketch of yourself dressed in your armor. Begin
your day praying on your armor. Then, you will most definitely
be equipped to withstand the schemes of the Devil.

March forward, my sweet soldier,
Mom

Dear Mom,

I may be clothed in spiritual armor, but this addiction makes
me feel naked. I have to strip down and look at the real me. It's
humiliating and painful.

It was fun to draw the sketch of myself in battle armor. Today, I'm concentrating on my helmet. That is, I'm reviewing the Bible verses and positive quotations that have helped the most. Then, I'm making a collage for my bulletin board. When I go into my office, I'll have a visual reminder of upbeat, positive guidance. And here I am, dressed in my Ephesians 6 armor:

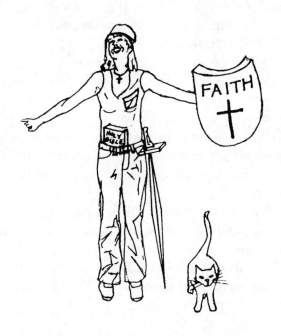

Smile Break

God will not look you over for medals, degrees, or diplomas, but for scars.

—Elbert Hubbard, *The Wisdom of the Midwest*

My Journal Page

Prayer

Almighty God, let Your power destroy my enemy today.

Action

Draw a sketch or visualize yourself dressed in God's armor (see Eph. 6:10–17).

To the Rescue

My dearest Kim,

Ever since you were a child, you've been compassionate and loving to animals. I think you were only four when our dog had a litter of twelve pups. What a time you had taking those puppies for a ride in your toy baby buggy.

As you grew older, you rescued the fallen and nursed to health the injured—you were Florence Nightingale with a wagon. Remember the baby sparrow that plummeted from its nest in the neighbor's tree? You scooped up the featherless blob, plopped it in your red wagon, and whisked it home. Then you shredded facial tissue, making a soft bed in a shoebox. For several days, you fed the nestling with an eyedropper. Despite your love, it died.

One of the cutest kittens we owned was Peanut, who had a magnificent tail that plumed in a fluffy arch. One day, Peanut appeared with his tail mangled. The vet had to amputate the broken tail and told us the cat had little chance of recovery. With your dedicated care and devotion, however, Peanut survived, but with only a stub as a reminder of his once-glorious tail.

I mention your love of your pets because I'm hoping you can direct some of that compassion to yourself. Be good to *you!*

Love,
Mom

Hello Mother,

You remember my success rescuing ill and injured cats and birds. But today I couldn't help my own pet. I had to say good-bye to Tigger. Remember how she came to us?

It was one icy Sunday ten years ago. We hadn't gone to church for several Sundays. Seldom did we go out the front door; we typically went through the garage. Rarely did we walk to church. But this day we walked out the front door to go across the street to church and I heard a kitten crying. I wanted to find that cat. Because we were late, I was urged to search when we got home.

All through the service I longed to find where the pitiful meows had come from. Back home, I put on my warmest clothes and pulled on my gloves. The earlier cries had seemed to emanate from our aboveground swimming pool that was covered for the winter. Digging through the folds of the pool cover, I found an almost frozen four-week-old kitten caked with ice in a crevice of the material. God had helped me find that kitten!

Cutting away a tangle of matted hair, I found Tigger. From her trauma, Tigger has always been afraid, hiding away under beds and in closets. Yet she has delighted us with her playfulness. For the past few months, however, she's been losing weight—the vet suspects an internal growth. Day by day, Tigger has grown weaker until all she can do is crawl to her water bowl and lie there with her head almost in the dish.

I couldn't bear to see Tigger in such misery. My heart was broken as I held her while the vet gave her an injection of anesthetic. Then I rocked her, stroked her, said good-bye to her, and left her to be euthanized. A cigarette would be a real comfort right now.

Grieving,

Kim

Smile Break

Most of us spend the first six days of each week sowing wild oats, then we go to church on Sunday and pray for a crop failure.

—Fred Allen

My Journal Page

Prayer

Divine Savior, rescue me from wanting to smoke today.

Action

Put a cigarette in a bottle of water. What do you think of the results?

_____

_____

_____

_____

_____

_____

_____

_____

_____

_____

_____

_____

_____

_____

_____

_____

_____

Grief with Glory

My sweet Kim,

It must be hard for you to lose Tigger—your trip to the vet was no doubt painful. Sometimes, I've found, the best of times accompany the worst of times. Sometimes glory comes with grief.

I remember how excited I was in April 1984 when I won my first writing awards in a statewide competition and how eager I was to tell Dad about my honors—except Dad was terminally ill with cancer, too weak to swallow a teaspoonful of water. Our town newspaper reported my five awards on the front page and printed my father's obituary on the back page.

When I lost my corporate job through downsizing, the hurt became bearable because your father and I had won a three-week trip on Amtrak. We boarded the train one week after my job of eleven years ended. We traveled by Superliner from Chicago and stopped in three places: San Antonio, Texas; Sacramento, California; and Portland, Oregon. As we sped along, I could enjoy the trip without stress—I would not have to return to my desk piled high with papers. And I wasn't squandering my precious vacation days on this trip. I was permanently on vacation!

Yes, happiness and heartache can be closely linked. I know a writer who told me that the joy of having her first book published was shadowed with sorrow. Two weeks before she held her book, ink-fresh from the printing press, her twenty-two-year-old son was killed in a mountain climbing accident.

I've wondered: Why does joy mix with sorrow? Perhaps it is to increase my faith. Perhaps it is to shape me into a more caring and understanding person. I do know that in peak times of joy and sharp pain, I've grown closer to God. Having experienced those heights and depths, I feel more compassion for others in their suffering.

In 2 Corinthians 1:3–4 it says, "Praise be to the God and Father of our Lord Jesus Christ, the Father of compassion and the God of all comfort, who comforts us in all our troubles, so that we can comfort those in any trouble with the comfort we ourselves have received from God." In your loss of your beloved kitten, I pray you'll glimpse some glory in your grief.

In sympathy,
Mom

Mother Dear,

As you reminded me of Grandpa Flora, I remembered a summer in my childhood when Grandpa and I were close. He had a large garden and I helped him pick green beans. Then we sat together under a shady maple and snapped those green beans. He was the grandpa who whistled, swinging his black metal lunch box as he walked up the drive coming home from his factory job. Happy to be home, he could then revel in the tomatoes, beets, and green beans in his well-tended garden.

Grandpa would be so sad to know I smoke. He would, on the other hand, be so happy to know I'd conquered a bad habit and quit smoking. It's been nineteen years since he was called home to heaven, but I remember him well. Such a godly man, always interested in each of us, his grandkids.

As for my grief over Tigger, I must let her go and remember the happy times.

Sadder but wiser,
Kim

Smile Break

There are two means of refuge from the miseries of life: music and cats.

—Albert Schweitzer

My Journal Page

Prayer

Dear Comforter, show me how to respond to others' sorrow.

Action

Do a kind deed for someone today.

_____

_____

_____

_____

_____

_____

_____

_____

_____

_____

_____

_____

_____

_____

_____

_____

_____

_____

———— *18* ————

Mighty Mouse Saves the Day

Dear Kim,

At the University of Dayton where I attended an Erma Bombeck workshop, I met Loretta LaRoche, who calls herself the Queen of Stress. Loretta is so funny she can make rocks giggle.

As keynote speaker, Loretta commented that many of us plan to enjoy ourselves the next week (after our weekend guests have left), or next year (after we've completed a big work project), or next decade (when we retire). She suggested we enjoy ourselves today—right now.

"What were women thinking," Loretta wondered, "when they passed up dessert before the Titanic sank?" And, she quipped, "Did you know stressed spelled backward is desserts?"

Loretta gave us tips on how to make each day a fun day by enjoying ourselves. We need to be as nutty as possible; need to have a good time; should keep our brains juicy; and should let go of being perfectionists.

She also told us to laugh every day. "Have you noticed children?" Loretta inquired. "A child of four laughs four hundred times a day!"

Relax, she said. Don't try to do everything for everyone—that makes you a martyr. Who wants her tombstone to read: "Did Everything—Died Anyway."

Be sure to exercise, she said. When working at a desk, get up and walk around; better yet, dance, or *twirl*. She explained, "Your computer crashes—you're stressed. Get up and twirl around."

For wacky fun, buy a blue satin Mighty Mouse cape. Loretta modeled hers and sang, "Here I've come to save the day—Mighty Mouse is on the way."

She suggested we could make a fashion statement by wearing an Attila the Hun hat sprouting two huge horns. She said, "Kids will love shopping in the mall with Mom wearing her Hun hat."

Think optimistically, Loretta declared. If you're asked, "How are you?" You should answer, "I'm so good I'm about to blow up!" Go around flinging your arms up and out, saying "Ta dah!" or "Whoopee!" Strut into a room and announce, "It's a good thing I'm here!"

Live abundantly and live creatively, she concluded. When you live abundantly, you flourish.

I'm reminded that her words echo those of Jesus, who said, "I have come that [you] may have life, and have it to the full" (John 10:10).

Lighten up and laugh,
Mom

Dear Mom,

I do need Mighty Mouse and a few laughs today. I've realized from my Freedom From Smoking class that people smoke for different reasons. Identifying those reasons is important. One of my reasons is that I reward myself with cigarettes. At my housecleaning job, when I finish cleaning a house, my reward is a smoke break.

If I get stressed, I reward myself with a cigarette.

As I start my day, I reward myself with a cup of coffee and a cigarette.

What I need to do is find another way to give myself a "treat." Because I enjoy my cats immensely, it may be something associated with them. Watching my cats playing and frolicking makes me laugh. Maybe I can sketch my kitties, or maybe I can videotape them. Finding substitute rewards deserves some more thought. . . .

Now that I've written this letter to you, I'm going to reward myself by watching a funny Loretta LaRoche video and smoking one—only one—cigarette.

Not!

That got your attention, didn't it? Oh, and considering my cats, I don't think I really should wear a Mighty *Mouse* cape.

Chuckling,
Kim

Smile Break

Time spent with cats is never wasted.

—Colette

My Journal Page

Prayer

Light of the World, thank You for the abundant life You've given me.

Action

Write down what makes you laugh. Identify the rewards you typically give yourself.

_____

_____

_____

_____

_____

_____

_____

_____

_____

_____

_____

_____

_____

_____

_____

_____

_____

19

Franklin Graham's Turning Point

Darling Kim,

In his book *Rebel with a Cause*,[1] Franklin Graham, the son of Billy and Ruth Graham, tells about his rebellion against God. In 1974, Franklin wrote, "the sinful life was not satisfying any longer. There was an emptiness—a big hole right in the middle of Franklin Graham's life. The truth was I felt miserable because my life wasn't right with God."

During a walk with his twenty-two-year-old son, Billy said, "Franklin, your mother and I sense there's a struggle going on in your life. You're going to have to make a choice either to accept Christ or reject Him. You can't continue to play the middle ground."

Soon after, Franklin chanced upon his friend David Hill, who was reading Romans 7 where Paul vividly describes the struggle with sin. David read this chapter aloud to Franklin. Listening, Franklin "broke out in a sweat and lit a cigarette to ease the tension. David didn't say another word at that moment—he just stared at me. I think he knew that God was speaking to me. I made some excuse to leave, but I couldn't forget the words David had just read. . . . I realized for the first time that sin had control over my life."

Franklin turned to Romans 8 and read, "There is therefore now no condemnation for those who are in Christ Jesus. . . . who do not walk according to the flesh, but according to the Spirit" (vv. 1, 4 NASB).

For several days he struggled. He read Romans 8:1 over and over. He writes, "I put my cigarette out and got down on my knees beside my bed. I'm not sure what I prayed, but I know that I poured out my heart to God and confessed my sin. I told Him I was sorry and that if He would take the pieces of my life and somehow put them back together, I was His. I wanted to live my life for Him from that day forward. I asked Him to forgive and cleanse me, and I invited Him by faith to come into my life."

That was Franklin's turning point. His years of running and rebellion had ended.

Praying for a turning point for you,
Mom

Dearest Mother,

I can relate to Franklin Graham's struggle, all right. You can't imagine how ashamed and guilty I feel because this addiction has me in its grip. There are times I want to avoid you and Dad because seeing you increases my guilt and shame big-time. I'm weary of being on the defensive.

When I can't sleep (and this is common), I read. One book written by Dr. Gerald G. May, titled *Addiction and Grace*,[2] has revealed some truths I've found helpful. Dr. May calls us to live lives of discernment, which means a prayerful life where one is as honest as possible with God and where one seeks God's guidance and then responds in faith. He writes, "A life lived this way, trying to bring all one's faculties into harmony with God's transforming grace is consecration in practice."

Although we want to think addictive behavior is complicated, Dr. May writes, it's really simple. "No matter how we might want to amplify and elaborate it, stopping addictive behavior boils down to this: Don't do it, refuse to do it, and keep refusing to do it. It is so simple, and it seems so impossible."

He goes on to say that our society has conditioned us to

think something is wrong with the way we're living if we feel distress, pain, deprivation, yearning, or longing. He says, "The truth is we were never meant to be completely satisfied." Dr. May points to Saint Augustine who said, "Our hearts will never rest, nor are they meant to rest, until they rest in God."

I think the bottom line is: I'm going to have pain. And I'm going to have to embrace two ugly words I've avoided: *I quit.*

With God's grace, there's hope for me,
Kim

Smile Break

Life is easier than you'd think; all that is necessary is to accept the impossible, do without the indispensable, and bear the intolerable.

—Kathleen Norris

My Journal Page

Prayer

Blessed Redeemer, thank You for not condemning me. Help me to live in Your Spirit and not in my flesh.

Action

Read and pray Romans 8:1, 4. What do these verses mean to you?

_____

_____

_____

_____

_____

_____

_____

_____

_____

_____

_____

_____

_____

_____

_____

_____

20

The Prayer of Power

Daughter Dear,

You said you liked to read about someone who is victorious after a struggle. Let me tell you how God helped me through a dark phase and how I took a giant spiritual step, discovering a powerful way to pray.

When I worked in corporate advertising, it was stressful. After nine fast-paced and frustrating years not being promoted or being able to change departments, I was very dissatisfied and felt like a failure. One day as I lunched by myself, reading a copy of *Guideposts*, a big tear fell on the page. Plip. Plop. Plip. Plop. One tear after another dropped. I ran out of the restaurant . . . sped home, and could not stop crying for a week! So began a long siege of clinical depression.

Slowly, I moved through a difficult year from darkness to light. I recall one summer day, during my lunch hour, as I sat sad and weary in my car in a shady park. Suddenly, I began praising God: "Thank you, Father, for this awful day. Thank you for what I'm learning about patience and suffering; and thank you I can sit at my desk instead of lying in my bed at home crying."

That change of heart, that shift to prayerful praise, helped me embrace my job with renewed vitality. Before long, I actually enjoyed my work! Then, when the company downsized me, I left knowing that God had new plans for me.

You, too, will come to realize that this wilderness experience culminates in spiritual growth. No matter how terrible the day gets, thank God for each struggle; thank him for how He's working in you. Today, sing along with your favorite CD of joy and praise.

As 1 Thessalonians 5:16–18 says, "Be joyful always; pray continually; give thanks in all circumstances, for this is God's will for you in Christ Jesus."

Praising Him,
Mom

My Mama,

Funny you should mention singing. John surprised me by giving me a tape called *Jesus*. The music is beautiful. There's nothing like a sing-along to keep my mind off a cigarette.

I bought $110 worth of nicotine patches. When John saw the sales receipt, he whistled (no tune involved).

Your telling me about the power of praising God in prayer inspired me to jot down blessings I'm thankful for. I praised God for each of these. Here's my list (in no special order):

1. Jesus
2. Mom
3. My husband, my daughter
4. My family
5. Cats and kittens
6. The earth's beauty
7. Health
8. Sunshine and all the seasons
9. A place of peace called Wheatfields
10. The Holy Spirit who guides me
11. Eternal life
12. Friends
13. Flowers
14. Banana taffy
15. Smiles
16. Seeing Christ in the faces of others

You know, Mom, your suffering through that depression was not for nothing—what you learned gives me a new perspective on prayer.

Pray on,
Kim

Smile Break

The most important prayer in the world is just two words long: "Thank you."

—Meister Eckhart

My Journal Page

Prayer

Holy God, thank You for stretching me. Thank You for the challenge of how to be grateful in each circumstance today.

Action

Describe how you feel as you sing along with your favorite CD of joy and praise.

_____

_____

_____

_____

_____

_____

_____

_____

_____

_____

_____

_____

_____

_____

_____

_____

21

Queenie Was a Meanie

Hi Kim,

When I was nine, I begged my father, "Please, Daddy, oh please, I want a pony of my very own." And my generous dad obliged. Queenie, a black Shetland pony with fat rounded sides, came to live with us.

When Dad was home, Queenie behaved. When Dad was gone, she showed her true character: ornery and stubborn. She'd puff out her sides when I saddled her, which led to dangerous consequences later. Queenie sensed my fear as I threw the saddle blanket over her broad back, cinched her saddle, and positioned the bridle between her huge teeth.

Queenie was a meanie. She purposely sidled under low tree branches, combing my hair and crowning me with bird nests. As a cowgirl, my riding style would have made Roy Rogers laugh; Dale Evans would have placed me at the top of her prayer list.

Everything spooked Queenie—a rock, a twig, a mud puddle. Seeing water, she'd snuff and snort and brake to a dead stop. Her fat body quivered under me like Jell-O. When she'd refuse to move, I'd urge her on with a click of my tongue. Queenie would take a fancy side step, tossing her head and mane. Then, without warning, she'd launch into a bouncy trot. *Wow-e-e-e-e!* By now the loose saddle had slipped, and I would be clamped to her side like human Velcro, yelling and screaming as we dodged bushes and telephone poles—and Queenie set a new speed record.

As time elapsed, I rode Queenie less and less. Dad replaced her with a submissive new bike that never rolled its eyes in terror or chomped me with horsey, yellow teeth. Queenie never learned to be submissive—something I find difficult to do, too. I stubbornly refuse to yield and surrender when God calls me to do the difficult. James 4:7 advises, "Submit yourselves, then, to God. Resist the devil, and he will flee from you."

With love,
Mom

Mother Dear,

I can't imagine you on a horse. You rode a pony! It sounds like Queenie was quite cantankerous. Looking back on bad days can be funny.

A favorite childhood book I read to Stephanie was Judith Viorst's *Alexander and the Terrible, Horrible, No Good, Very Bad Day*. Alexander experiences a disappointment at breakfast, a bad seat in the car riding to school, rejection from his teacher, and a visit to the dentist. His solution to his problems is typical—wanting to escape. As he considers each trouble, he chirps, "I want to go to Australia."

Viorst's book parallels how overwhelmed I was today. I craved a cigarette like a fish needs water. My nicotine patch was on; I'd prayed and put on my full armor; but my arm holding up the great shield of faith to ward off the arrows of the evil one turned to rubber. I grew weak.

Then an amazing thing happened. Kathy and Mike walked in the door with a surprise. They'd found a stray kitty—a puff of gray fluff. He must be only three weeks old but very brave. Twice he crossed State Road 9 to get to Mike and Kathy. I don't know why he wasn't killed.

Taking care of this orphan took my mind off wanting a cigarette. Then Grandma Pearl arrived with a fresh-baked blackberry pie. So, my terrible, horrible, no good, very bad day changed when four angels came on missions of mercy.

And I don't have to go to Australia.

Surviving,
Kim

Smile Break

Courage is being scared to death and saddling up anyway.

—John Wayne, *The Wisdom of the Midwest*

My Journal Page

Prayer

Abba Father, help me to be pliable, not stubborn.

Action

Reflect on where you need to be submissive.

_____

_____

_____

_____

_____

_____

_____

_____

_____

_____

_____

_____

_____

_____

_____

_____

First Place in My Life

Dear Kim,

When you study God's Word, He is gracious to show you the truths He wants you to know. About twenty years ago, my faith walk took a quantum leap forward when I learned the importance of Matthew 22:36–38. Jesus was asked, "Teacher, which is the greatest commandment in the Law?"

He replied, "Love the Lord your God with all your heart and with all your soul and with all your mind. This is the first and greatest commandment."

When I considered these verses, I realized that someone else held first place in my heart. My husband (your dad); and my children—you, Kathy, and Kerry. My life centered around the four of you.

So I had to surrender my precious four loved ones to God and let Him be first and utmost. This is hard to do—but essential.

Who holds first place in your life? Your daughter? Your husband? Your kitties? Your art? Examine your heart; then choose to place God as your *number-one first priority.* It will truly make a difference.

As you surrender your all to God, may you enjoy the peace that passes all understanding.

My love,
Mom

Dear Mom,

Sadly—I hate to admit this, but being honest—cigarettes have been *number one* in my life. They are typically my first thought in the morning. I wouldn't consider going anyplace without a cigarette. Truth be told, I do put Stephanie, John, and my cats high on my list of priorities. But this is the first time I've pondered this question: Who is *first* in my life?

I know Jesus is working on me. If I'm not wearing the patch and I do smoke a cigarette, it's not very pleasurable. Each time I stumble, rip off my patch, and smoke, I'm overcome with remorse and shame. My desire is waning. Why do I hang on to this guilt and shame?

God has a sense of humor. I've taken the next step from smoking in the dark, dingy basement. Now I inconvenience myself further by going totally *outside* the house. Where do I sneak a smoke when I take off the patch? I smoke on the front porch as I sit in our new swing!

The other night, while relaxing in the swing, I decided I'd been very good. Proud of myself, I decided to allow myself one cigarette. As the smoke curled around my head, I looked across the street at the church. There was an opening in the full, leafy branches of the surrounding trees, and one thing was highlighted in the open space. What did I see? There, all lit up, was the shining stained glass window—the Lamb of God who takes away the sin of the world.

How ironic! God is shining His light in my darkness, and I can't escape this truth. I see how ludicrous this whole thing is. It's funny. I wonder what it will take? How much more affirmation do I need to realize the Lord's will for me? There is no doubt! This is hard—when His will and truth are known—I cannot run away. It is there in my face, with the light shining on it.

Hoping for illumination,
Kim

Smile Break

Hope itself is like a star—not to be seen in the sunshine of prosperity, and only discovered in the night of adversity.

—Charles Spurgeon

My Journal Page

Prayer

Sovereign Lord, I surrender my precious "loves" to You. You hold the most honored first place in my heart and soul.

Action

Take a prayer walk. Jot down what you've learned.

_____

_____

_____

_____

_____

_____

_____

_____

_____

_____

_____

_____

_____

_____

_____

_____

_____

23

Seeking Silence

Sweetest Kim,

There are eight words in Psalms 46:10 that I find hard to follow: "Be still, and know that I am God."

Silence is a rare commodity. Even at 6 A.M. in my sleepy house, noises abound. Our refrigerator hums, then the ice maker clunks out ice cubes. An airplane mumbles across the sky outside. A block away, on State Road 9, a truck rumbles along.

Yet Isaiah 30:15 notes, "This is what the Sovereign LORD, the Holy One of Israel, says: 'In repentance and rest is your salvation, in *quietness* and trust is your strength'" (emphasis mine).

This week, if possible, set aside quiet time to be with God. This silence will strengthen and uplift you.

Mother Teresa said, "We need to find God and he cannot be found in noise and restlessness. God is the friend of silence. See how nature—trees, flowers, grass—grows in silence. The essential thing is not what we say, but what God says to us and through us. All our words will be useless unless they come from within; words that do not give the light of Christ increase the darkness."[1]

Seek silence with Him.

Lovingly,
Mom

Dear Mom,

Seeking silence, I went to Wheatfields, the natural arts learning center near home. Its gardens and nature trails are a refuge for me. Maybe Bluebell, their resident hawk, might dip his wings at me as he soars over the trees.

On my drive to Wheatfields, I sang songs of praise. As I approached the red farmhouse and old barn, I looked in the sky. I couldn't believe what I saw. Clouds had formed a large smile in the sky. God blessed me with a smiley face—it was a boost I needed.

Thank You, Lord, for the strength to resist smoking this day. Thank You for smiling on me. Thank You for our quiet time together.

Awed by an awesome God,
Kim

Smile Break

A smile is a curve that sets everything straight.
—Phyllis Diller

My Journal Page

Prayer

Most Holy One, help me to be still and know that You are God.

Action

Find quiet time to be alone with God.

_____

_____

_____

_____

_____

_____

_____

_____

_____

_____

_____

_____

_____

_____

_____

_____

_____

_____

_____

_____

24

What Elvis Presley Taught Me

Dear Kim,

Not many can claim they have Elvis Presley living with them—but I can. At a fund-raising auction, I won the bid on Elvis. Yes, he's a life-size cardboard cutout, and this Elvis talks (with a battery-activated sensor). Dressed in a gold tuxedo with gold shoes, Elvis (all six feet of him) stands like a sentinel in the corner of my bedroom.

As a teenager, I remember playing my 45 rpm records of "You Ain't Nothin' but a Hound Dog" until they lost their grooves and my parents wanted to stomp on my "Blue Suede Shoes." What saddened me was watching Elvis perform his last TV concert. My teen idol had grown portly, and he sweated profusely as he sang "I Did It My Way."

As I walk by my cardboard King of Rock and Roll, he chirps, "Hi, this is Elvis Presley." When I open the drawer for clean socks, he croons, "Honey, you can have anything I've got." If a button pops off my slacks, Elvis assures me it's "no big deal."

When Elvis died August 16, 1977, he'd already sold one billion records. He was fabulously rich. However, "King" Elvis was also miserable and lonely—he'd never attained peace. Actually, he makes me think of King Solomon, who had great riches but let seven hundred pagan wives woo him to worship idols. He did evil in the eyes of the Lord.

"When I surveyed all that my hands had done and what I had toiled to achieve," Solomon lamented, "everything was meaningless, a chasing after the wind; nothing was gained under the sun" (Eccl. 2:11).

The Elvis in my bedroom reminds me that fame is fleeting; wealth doesn't bring happiness, and living "My Way" leads to self-destruction. The other day, I said to Elvis, "You know, King Solomon in Ecclesiastes 12:13 finally got it right; he declared, 'Fear God and keep his commandments, for this is the whole duty of man.'"

His dark eyes smoldering, Elvis replied, "Thank you. Thank you very much."

Consider what is meaningless in your life.

Love,
Mom

Mother, Mother,

Instead of what's meaningless—let me turn that around and remember the tips and techniques that have been *meaningful* and helped me:

- Having an oral substitute—that is, something in my hand instead of a cigarette. I cut plastic drinking straws in half and puffed on them.
- Carrying bottled water with me instead of cigarettes.
- Doing something with my hands—such as organizing the kitchen cabinets, rearranging furniture, or working a jig-saw puzzle.
- Taking breaks during housecleaning by stepping outside and taking deep breaths.
- Rewarding myself with a professional haircut. (I normally hack away at my own hair.)
- Taking walks.

Remember now, "Love Me Tender,"
Kim

Smile Break

What can you say about a society that says that God is dead and Elvis is still alive?

—Irv Kupcinet

My Journal Page

Prayer

Holy Spirit, help me to be pliable, to strongly desire to live "Your Way."

Action

Remember the tips and techniques that have been *meaningful* and helped you.

_____

_____

_____

_____

_____

_____

_____

_____

_____

_____

_____

_____

_____

_____

_____

_____

_____

_____

25

Zero Tolerance

Hi Kim,

A new study may show why smokers so easily return to the habit even years after they quit. The key may be tolerance to nicotine, say researchers at the University of Pittsburgh School of Medicine. "Tolerance . . . can explain why someone can rapidly go back to a pack a day, even after not smoking for a long time," says study author Dr. Kenneth Perkins, a professor of psychiatry at Pittsburgh.

Perkins says that most people don't get hooked on cigarettes when they first start smoking because their tolerance to nicotine is low. "They can smoke a few cigarettes, feel satisfied, and not have to smoke any more."

However, the longer you smoke, he says, the more tolerant you become to nicotine's effects. It takes more and more cigarettes to give the same feeling of satisfaction. A new study reported in the November 2001 issue of the journal *Psychopharmacology* shows that once a person is hooked on smoking, tolerance to nicotine never declines, even years after not smoking. Should one go back to smoking, this sustained elevation allows the person to develop a full-blown habit much faster than when the person first started to smoke.

"We did not expect the tolerance levels to nicotine to be so permanent. It shows that once you become hooked on cigarettes, your response to nicotine can never return to the pre-smoking state," Perkins notes. He continues, "If you are lucky enough to have successfully quit, don't kid yourself into thinking you can resume a 'casual' habit. With brain chemistry already 'pre-wired' to smoke, it may not take much for your old habit to kick in."[1]

So, don't fool yourself, Kim. You have zero tolerance to nicotine. It may take only one cigarette, and you're hooked again. It's a harsh reality, but you need to know the truth. Jesus said in John 8:31–32, "If you hold to my teaching, you are really my disciples. Then you will know the truth, and the truth will set you free."

Let the truth of this research impress upon you the danger of smoking even one more cigarette.

Love always,
Mom

Dear Mom,

You're right, Mom. Whenever I've attempted to quit before, my downfall has related to two things. I've not leaned on the Holy Spirit. And I've convinced myself that I've conquered my addiction and it's safe to smoke that one cigarette.

I learned from a health article on the Internet that most people try to quit smoking five to seven times before they're successful. The article also said that smokers need to be aware they're making a long-term commitment, and the longer they can stay off cigarettes, the better their chance for success.

I must have tried to stop five or six times. I've read that stopping smoking is like a revolving door. Many smokers go around several times before leaving it. The rotation includes preparing to stop, stopping, and relapsing. The article said, "If you don't stop the first time you try, try again. Eventually you will succeed."

I'm getting dizzy, going around. . . .

Ready to shoot out the door,
Kim

Smile Break

Heavenly Father, hear my plea
And grant my lungs serenity!
Give me strength to kick the smoking
That's been causing all my choking.

Let my breath be fresh and clean,
Without a trace of nicotine.
Guide me by your holy means,
Past all cigarette machines.

I ask your help,
And it's no wonder
If I don't quit,
I'm six feet under!
Amen.

—Author Unknown

My Journal Page

Prayer

Holy Spirit, brand the words *zero tolerance* on my mind.

Action

Make a wallet card that says, "Warning: One Cigarette Always Leads to Another."

26

God's Plan for Your Life

My Dear Kim,

Have you ever asked, "What is God's plan for my life?" That question burned within me for years. Although I struggled and prayed, I wasn't sure what my mission in life was. Then, as I once again questioned the Lord, "What am I to do for you?" it seemed as if a voice said, "You don't have to *do* anything, just *be.*"

What comforting words! God wants me not to *do* great things for Him but to *be* with Him. Soon after that revelation, I attended a retreat at the Abbey of Gethsemani near Bardstown, Kentucky. This retreat focused on silence and journaling. As we sat in a circle on the floor, writing, our instructor placed an object on the floor in the center of the circle. It was a white coffee mug. As I looked at that pure white cup, I knew I wanted to be like it: clean and empty so the Lord could fill me with His love.

As I spent quiet time listening to God, studying Scripture, and praying, He *did* reveal what He wants me to do. The time spent alone with Him was preparation.

Kim, as you search for God's plan for you, remember that He cherishes time with you. God may not want you to *do* anything but just *be* with Him. At the right time you will know, most assuredly, what God wants you to do. You can find assurance in Jeremiah 29:11: "'For I know the plans I have for you,' declares the Lord, 'plans to prosper you and not to harm you, plans to give you hope and a future.'"

Excited about His plan for you,
Mom

My Mama,

I did set aside some quiet time today to be with God. It shouldn't be just a one-day occurrence, I know. God's plan for me may be to use me as a witness. However, in my heart, I realize I can't be an effective witness if I'm puffing smoke like a tugboat.

When I go to church and social events, I'm ashamed because I smell like an ashtray. I try to distance myself from others and sit in the balcony. This addiction makes me very ashamed. Cravings come during the service, and I want to hurry to the parking lot and light up.

Right now, I don't know what God's plan is for me. Maybe I need to concentrate on my art talent. Sculpture has been my favorite medium. Sculpting is a joy. At a local art fair this weekend, I met a sculptor who works with alabaster. It was fascinating to talk to him, and I got excited thinking about taking a class he teaches. One thing about it—if I'm sculpting, I don't have a free hand to hold a cigarette.

Keep me in your prayers,
Kim

Smile Break

Usually we trust that nature has a master plan. But what was it she expected to do with tobacco?

—Bill Vaughan,
Kansas City Star

My Journal Page

Prayer

Abba Father, I seek Your will for my life. Open my eyes that I might see Your plan for me. Quiet my soul so I can be a white, empty cup filled with Your love and peace.

Action

Don't *do*, just *be* with God for a while today.

27

The Long Haul

My Dear Kim,

Each of us has a weakness that allows Satan to disable us. For me, it's discouragement. When I get a rejection letter from an editor, I'm devastated. Next, self-doubt creeps in. I think if I've been rejected it must mean I'll never have another creative idea; all my time invested was a waste; I'm a failure. The downward spiral puts me in the dumps, and the devil has successfully sidetracked me from my writing goal.

Whenever discouragement grips you, get a grip! You may hit a pothole; you may really be disheartened. You may want to quit this whole thing, but you hate to let me down and disappoint me. Hey, I'm here for the *long haul.* Even if it takes six months, even if it takes a year, keep trying. Let's keep on *truckin'!*

We've embarked on the road to smoke-free living, and no matter how many detours, we're rolling on. Jeremiah 31:21 says, "Set up road signs; put up guideposts. Take note of the highway, the road that you take."

We're truckin' on the road to success.

Cheerio,
Mom

Dear Mom,

Every day I get more prepared for the long haul. Thank you, Mom, for being my sidekick, my relief driver in our big ol' truck.

I've come to some lightbulb moments in the last few weeks.

Getting to know who I really am, getting to know my genuine self.

For my birthday, Grandma Pearl gave me a fantastic book, *Self Matters* by Dr. Phil. I stayed up until 4 A.M. reading it this morning. Have you and Dr. Phil been collaborating? What he says, what you have written, and what I've learned from Bible study have come together in some major revelations.

Dr. Phil says that if I'm not living my passion, my life has no purpose. I know that my passions are God, art, my health, and being able to help others. When I get my arms around all of those, and live accordingly, I don't think cigarettes are going to mean much to me.

I've loved your letters, Mom, because they direct me to the truth—the truth of God's Word and His love for me. The truth about my purpose here on earth.

I'm excited about getting to know Jesus more intimately each day. I'm excited about studying sculpting with alabaster. I'm excited about using my cats in my artwork. And, I'm excited because I want to stop smoking for me—not for you, not for Dad, not for Stephanie, not for John, but for me.

I'm mapping my route,
Kim

Smile Break

The road to success is always under construction.
—Lily Tomlin, *The Funny Pages*

My Journal Page

Prayer

God of Glory, You rule over heaven and earth, highway and home. Fuel me with Your faith; steady me when the road gets bumpy.

Action

Take a drive along a scenic route. Describe how earth's beauty affects you.

_____

_____

_____

_____

_____

_____

_____

_____

_____

_____

_____

_____

_____

_____

_____

_____

28

Carol Burnett and Daughter Carrie

Precious Daughter,

You've mentioned before that you want to quit smoking—to live for the sake of your daughter, Stephanie. This reminded me of the time when Barbara Walters interviewed Carol Burnett about her relationship with her daughter Carrie Hamilton.[1] I thought of us. Carol and Carrie enjoyed collaborating on a special project, just as you and I have worked together on this book.

Do you remember Carol Burnett's reign as queen of television comedy during the 1970s? She closed each show with a song and her trademark good-night gesture—a gentle tug on her ear. It was a secret way of saying "Hello, I love you" to her grandmother, Nanny, who raised her.

Carol's three daughters, Carrie, Jody, and Erin Hamilton, practically grew up on the set of Carol's weekly show. When Carrie was thirteen, Carol was shocked to learn that her eldest was heavily addicted to drugs and alcohol. With Carol's help, Carrie won a four-year battle over the addictions; mother and daughter became closer than ever.

When Carrie wrote a play based on her mother's 1986 autobiography, *One More Time,* Carol gained new respect for her daughter as a writer. They worked as equals on this special project. Then August 2001 brought dreaded news—Carrie, a longtime smoker, was diagnosed with lung cancer. While she underwent chemotherapy and radiation, she kept her sense of humor even as she lost her hair.

"Carrie had a spirit about her, all through her treatments,"

Carol said. When Carrie had a relapse and returned to the hospital, she told her mom she'd "missed the food." "We both started to howl," Carol said.

Much as Carrie hoped to triumph over cancer, she learned in November 2001 that her lung cancer had spread to her brain. In her last weeks, Carrie helped her mother in casting decisions for the play *Hollywood Arms.*

In long talks about the rough years, Carrie apologized to her mom for smoking. On January 20, 2002, Carrie Hamilton died. She was thirty-eight. *Hollywood Arms* opened to positive reviews in Chicago three months later. It was, Carol believes, Carrie's legacy. Carol said that she still says good night to audiences with a tug on her ear, but now she's doing it for Nanny *and* for Carrie.

I thank God we can continue to collaborate on our book.

Blessed to still have you,
Mom

Dearest Mother,
I cried a bucket after reading about Carol Burnett and Carrie. I can identify with Carrie's struggles so much. I, too, have battled on and off for four years to give up this addiction. It's been painful, but I have learned much about my Savior and about myself. His truths, accompanied by His love and your love, have made me stronger. I can feel God's strength and presence around me and in me.

It's time for me to take another step. I don't want our story to end like Carol's and Carrie's. I want to live many healthy years glorifying my Jesus. Yes, I know my physical body has been pushed to the limit. It can't take another year of smoking. I'm ready to claim my victory and for the battle to cease.

My actions . . . I'm falling to my knees and asking for a miracle and God's mercies. I'll continue to wear my patch. I will remain in Bible study, trusting God. I'll wear my mustard seed necklace you gave me because it reminds me to have faith and believe that miracles happen.

It has been four years since I created any art. I miss it tremendously. What good is an artist who doesn't create? I've been cheating myself far too long. I want my artist's voice back, but this time with no smoke in my throat. If I focus on Jesus and my art, I'm confident a miracle will come. This worked for me when I battled depression twelve years ago.

Mom, I assure you I am *never giving up!* Because winners never quit. I will do whatever it takes.

Winning with Christ,
Kim

Smile Break

Grief can take care of itself, but to get the full value of joy, you must have someone to divide it with.

—Mark Twain

My Journal Page

Prayer

Gentle Shepherd, thank You for each moment with my loved ones.

Action

Tell about a special time you've had with those you love.

_____

_____

_____

_____

_____

_____

_____

_____

_____

_____

_____

_____

_____

_____

_____

_____

_____

_____

Making a Commitment

Dearest Kim,

According to an article in *The Indianapolis Star,* commitment is the key to quitting smoking. When University of Wisconsin-Madison physician Michael Fiore talks about ending addiction to tobacco, people notice. Dr. Fiore leads a multimillion-dollar research project designed to learn why people have trouble stopping smoking and how to help them.

"I am convinced that everyone who smokes, if committed . . . can quit," Dr. Fiore claims.

In 1997, 48 million adults smoked. About 20 million adults will try to quit smoking. Dr. Fiore says, "While tobacco is a powerfully addictive substance, commitment and clinical assistance can result in most smokers successfully quitting. But until a person makes a decision to stop smoking, it won't happen."[1]

Commitment, Kim, is a hard word to embrace—it means not giving up. It means going on even if there are setbacks; it means keeping the faith.

Psalm 37:5–6 tells us, "Commit your way to the Lord; trust in him and he will do this: He will make your righteousness shine like the dawn, the justice of your cause like the noonday sun."

Much love,
Mom

Dear Mom,

    This is it! I'm making a commitment today to stop smoking. You can be my witness and sign your name.

> I, Kim Nading, do covenant and commit not to smoke
> for 60 days.

> Witnessed by: Jean Flora Glick
> Date: October 3, 2002

    I want a record of my successes, so I'm hanging a big calendar on the wall. Every day that I'm smoke free, I'll add a smiley face sticker to that day on the calendar. I guess I'm like a school kid who wants to earn a star from the teacher.

    If smiley face stickers aren't enough to keep me to my commitment, there is one other option—you might offer me a bribe! Maybe a Mercedes-Benz or a trip to Europe?

Just kidding,
Kim

Smile Break

Character consists of what you do on the third and fourth tries.

—James Michener, *Chesapeake*

My Journal Page

Prayer

Unchangeable God, I want to make a commitment—trusting in You, believing You will help me to quit smoking.

Action

Sign a covenant, when you are really ready.

I, _____ , do covenant and commit
   (your name)

not to smoke for _____ days.

Witnessed by: _____
Date: _____

_____ *30* _____

Your Friend, the Cigarette

Hi Kim,

For all these years, you've cherished your relationship with your companion, the Cigarette. Check out this excerpt from an article titled "My Cigarette, My Friend" that I found on an Internet Web site:

> How do you feel about a friend who has to go everywhere with you? Not only does he tag along all the time, but since he is so offensive and vulgar, you become unwelcome when with him. He has a peculiar odor that sticks to you wherever you go. Others think both of you stink.
>
> He controls you totally. When he says jump, you jump. Sometimes in the middle of a blizzard or storm, he wants you to come to the store and pick him up. . . . Sometimes, when you are out at a movie or play, he says he wants you to go stand in the lobby with him and miss important scenes. Since he calls all the shots in your life, you go.
>
> Your friend doesn't like your choice of clothing, either. Instead of politely telling you that you have lousy taste, he burns little holes in these itcms so you will want to throw them out. Sometimes he tires of the furniture and gets rid of it, too. Occasionally he gets really nasty and decides the whole house must go.

He gets pretty expensive to support. Not only is his knack of property destruction costly, but you must pay to keep him with you. In fact, he will cost you thousands of dollars over your lifetime. And you can count on one thing; he will never pay you a penny in return.

Often at picnics you watch others playing vigorous activities and having lots of fun doing them. But your friend won't let you. He doesn't believe in physical activity. In his opinion, you are too old to have that kind of fun. So he kind of sits on your chest and makes it difficult for you to breathe. Now, you don't want to go off and play with other people when you can't breathe, do you?

Your friend does not believe in being healthy. He is really repulsed by the thought of you living a long and productive life. So every chance he gets, he makes you sick. He helps you catch colds and flu. Not just by running out in the middle of the lousy weather to pick him up at the store. He is more creative than that. He carries thousands of poisons with him, which he constantly blows in your face. When you inhale some of them, they wipe out cilia in your lungs that would have helped you prevent these diseases.

But colds and flu are just his form of child's play. He especially likes diseases that slowly cripple you—like emphysema. He considers this disease great. Once he gets you to have this, you will give up all your other friends, family, career goals, activities—everything. You will just sit home and caress him, telling him what a great friend he is while you desperately gasp for air.

But eventually your friend tires of you. He decides he no longer wishes to have your company. Instead of letting you go your separate ways, he decides to kill you. He has a wonderful arsenal of weapons behind him. In fact, he has been plotting your death since the day you met him. He picked all the top killers in society and did everything in his power to ensure you would get one of them. He overworked your heart and lungs. He clogged up the arteries to your heart, brain, and every other part of your body. In case you were too strong to succumb to this, he constantly exposed you to cancer-causing agents. He knew he would get you sooner or later.

Well, this is the story of your "friend," your cigarette. No real friend would do all this to you. Cigarettes are the worst possible enemies you ever had. They are expensive, addictive, socially unacceptable, and deadly. Consider all this and—NEVER TAKE ANOTHER PUFF![1]

Is the Cigarette your friend, Kim? Proverbs 17:17 says, "A friend loves at all times. . . ." Can you say that about your buddy, the Cigarette?

Knowing who your True Friend is,
Mom

Dear Mom,
This is my letter to my friend, the Cigarette:

I thought you were my friend, but now I know that

you are the great deceiver. I believed you when you told me we deserved each other. I believed you when you told me you were the only one who could comfort me. I believed you when you convinced me that you would not hurt me. I believed you when you told me it was impossible to leave you.

I thought you were my friend, but now I know that you are the great thief. Little by little you took my self-confidence and self-esteem. You robbed me of my dignity. Puff by puff you stole my energy, my health, and my zest for life. You even tried to take my soul, but that was already spoken for.

I thought you were my friend, but now I know that you are my greatest enemy. Puff by puff you made me an addict. Puff by puff I became more isolated and more withdrawn. Puff by puff I became your slave and you became my master. Every minute of my life was centered around you.

I thought you were my friend—until my real friend, Jesus, opened my eyes and removed your smoke screen. I thought you were my friend—until my real friend, Jesus, convicted me and shed His light on your darkness. When my real friend, Jesus, came calling again, I realized how much I missed Him and how much I needed Him.

My real friend, Jesus, told me it was time to make a choice. I had to choose who would be my master. I chose Jesus. There's no room for you now or evermore. So go, walk out the door. I don't need you anymore. Jesus came to save me from your bondage and set me free. So go, you won't deceive me or rob me any longer. Jesus is my strength, and all things are possible through God who strengthens me.

Smile Break

A friend comes in when the whole world goes out.
                                    —Anonymous

My Journal Page

Prayer

Lord Jesus, thank You for being my Forever Friend.

Action

Write a letter to your friend, the Cigarette.

_____

_____

_____

_____

_____

_____

_____

_____

_____

_____

_____

_____

_____

_____

_____

_____

_____

_____

Kim's Epilogue

Dear Reader,

If there's one thing I want you to know, it's this: I could not quit smoking without God's help. Overcoming a nicotine addiction is not something I could do of my own human will. I did make a commitment and set an "I Quit Day." Yes, there has been a victory in Jesus—I've quit smoking for sixty days. (Lots of smiley faces on my calendar.)

Your journey and my journey will be different, but I pray that with the help of the Holy Spirit, you can stop smoking too.

If I do let my guard down and—I hate this thought—start smoking again, I know I can begin again to quit again. With God there is always hope.

> "May the God of hope fill you with all joy and peace as you trust in him, so that you may overflow with hope by the power of the Holy Spirit" (Rom. 15:13).

You can do it!

Kim

P.S. E-mail me with your victories at holysmokes@kregel.com.

Smile Break

Hope is the thing with feathers,
That perches in the soul
And sings the tunes without the words
And never stops at all.

—Emily Dickinson

Endnotes

Chapter 11: Benefits of Not Smoking
1. American Lung Association. http://wwwquitsmokingnews.com/index.shtml.

Chapter 14: Kissable Lips
1. http://www.niconews.com/RLibrary/yet_another.htm.

Chapter 19: Franklin Graham's Turning Point
1. Franklin Graham, *Rebel with a Cause* (Nashville: Thomas Nelson, Inc., 1995), excerpts from pages 119–125.
2. Gerald G. May, *Addiction and Grace* (San Francisco: Harper & Row, 1988), 177–80.

Chapter 23: Seeking Silence
1. Mother Teresa, *A Gift for God: Prayers and Meditations* (New York: Harper San Francisco, 1996), 68–69.

Chapter 25: Zero Tolerance
1. Colette Bouchez, "Study Explains Ex-Smokers' Ever-Burning Desire." http://www.no-smoking.org/nov01/11-16-01-4.html.

Chapter 28: Carol Burnett and Daughter Carrie
1. http.//more.abcnews.go.com/sections/2020/DailyNews/2020_burnett_020614.html.

Chapter 29: Making a Commitment
1. Lawanza L. Griffin, "Commitment to quitting is primary, researcher-doctor says," *The Indianapolis Star,* 23 April 2000, J5.

Chapter 30: Your Friend, the Cigarette
1. Adapted from "My Cigarette, My Friend," by Joel Spitzer, © 1984, 2000. Used by permission. All rights reserved. First

published in *Respiratory Tract,* the official publication of the Illinois Society for Respiratory Therapy, vol. 11, no. 1 (January 1985). Full article can be found online at http://www.whyquit.com/joel/Joel_02_01_my_cig_my_friend.html.

Resources

Franklin Graham, *Rebel with a Cause* (Nashville: Thomas Nelson, Inc., 1995).

Loretta LaRoche, *Relax–You May Only Have a Few Minutes Left* (New York: Villard, 1998). Web site: www.lorettalaroche.com.

Gerald G. May, *Addiction and Grace* (San Francisco: Harper & Row, 1988).

Phillip C. McGraw, *Self Matters* (New York: Simon and Schuster Source, 2001).

Charles Stanley, *The Wonderful Spirit-Filled Life* (Nashville: Oliver–Nelson, 1992).